NZ Iron Level 1 Training Manual

Darryl Grauman

Photos by: Dieneké Erazzo

Additional Text by: Aimee Kovacevic

Darryl Grauman

ISBN:
ISBN-13: 978-1974036585

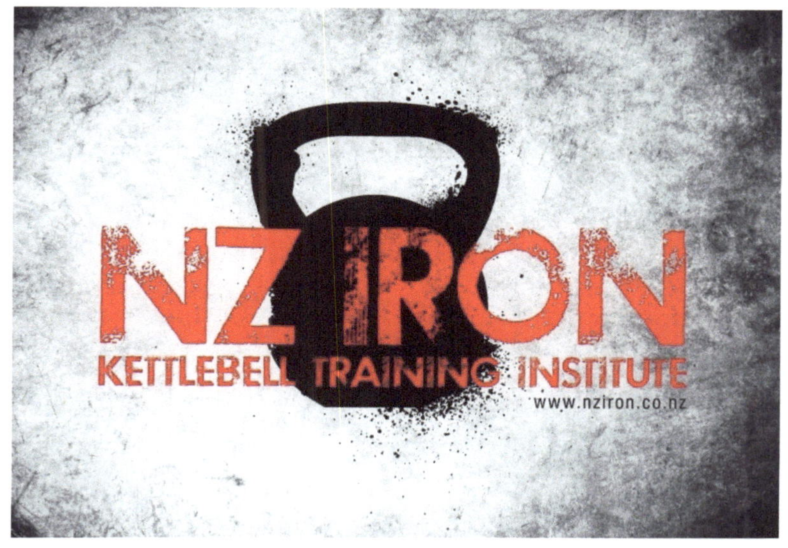

Kettlebell Training Manual

Darryl Grauman

NZ IRON

Functional Movement Basic and Intermediate Training Manual

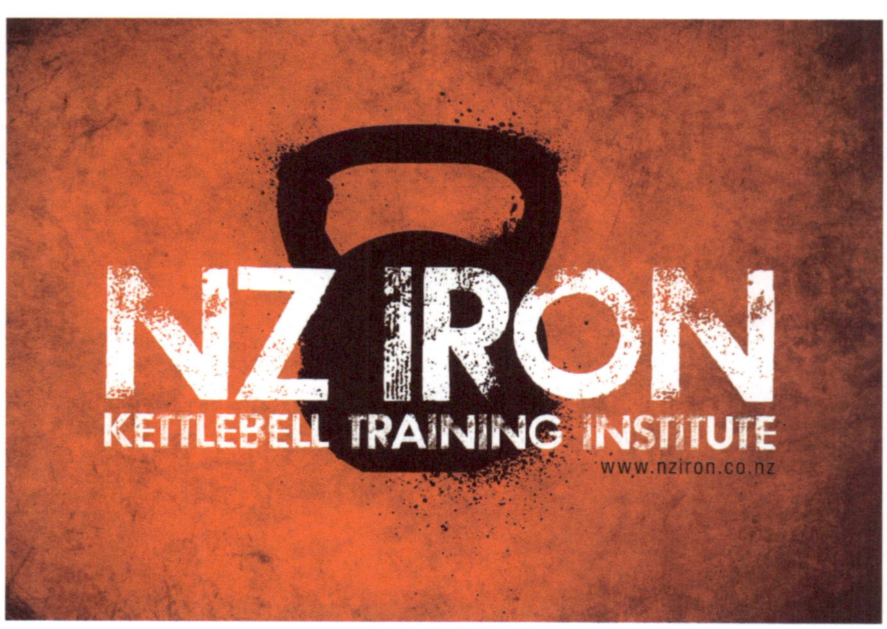

Foreword

The NZ Iron organisation was created specifically to teach fitness enthusiasts as well as exercise professionals and physical therapists the correct and most beneficial way to use kettlebells. A kettlebell can be dangerous in the hands of an untrained person. Swinging large metal weights the wrong way, can cause more harm than good.

This manual started out as a companion to the NZ Iron Level 1 Kettlebell Course. Through the evolution of NZ Iron, our students and social media, this text has evolved into a stand-alone manual.

Remember that a good cookbook does not make a Master Chef, and although I have read many books on anatomy, I've never once attempted surgery – therefore this text is also not a substitute for a course where professional instructors can correct both form as well as teaching methods. We cannot stress the importance of a good teacher.

My Kettlebell teacher, Dr Mark Cheng (who's bio I have included in the back of this text and is to this day one of the world's leading experts in human performance training) was key to my understanding of technique, strength training, rehabilitative and preventative practices through the use of kettlebells. Nothing can substitute a good teacher!

I hope that with this text as an additional reference, your kettlebell training progresses from strength to strength.

<u>Our Schedule for this 2-day course:</u>

<u>Day 1:</u>

1. What is a Kettlebell?
2. KBs for Pre-habilitation, rehabilitation, strength, fitness, weight loss.
3. What is "Functional Movement"
4. MVO2
5. The "Central Governor" Theory
6. Techniques:
    a. Deadlift
    b. Goblet Squat
    c. Swing
    d. Clean
    e. Bicep Curl
7. <u>Day 1 Class</u>: Group Workout
8. Q & A

<u>Day 2:</u>

1. Day 1 Recap
2. Techniques:
    a. Clean & Press
    b. 1-Arm Swing
    c. Alternating Swing
    d. Snatch
    e. Military Press
    f. 2-Hand Upright Row
    g. Turkish Get-Up
3. <u>Day 2 Class</u>: Group Workout
4. Exam Prep
5. Q & A

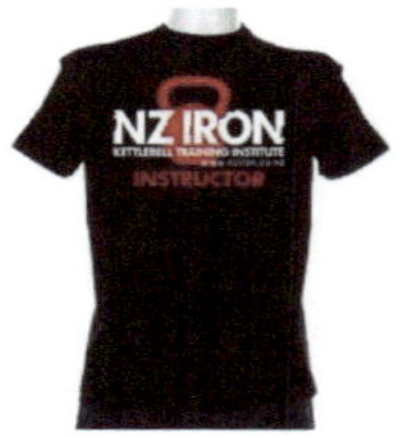

INTRODUCTION

What is a Kettlebell?

A Kettlebell is like a bowling ball with a thick shaped handle. The off-centred nature of the weight makes training with it difficult if you lack the proper form. Unlike bodybuilding style workouts which focus all the stress on a single muscle group, Kettlebell style training recruits many different muscle groups at the same time. This trains you to use your body synergistically, moving as a coordinated whole. Thus, a Kettlebell, when used properly, develops functional movement, strength, flexibility AND cardio all at the same time. Slowly but surely, in addition to strength and conditioning training, the Kettlebell is becoming a recognised too for rehabilitative and pre-habilitative training.

What Kettlebells do for you
(health effects)

A Kettlebell on its own does nothing, especially if it is left on the floor and you stare at it from time-to-time. What is important is how you lift it, how you swing it, how frequently, how fast (or slow) and how many times you use it. Kettlebells, if done correctly, will assist you to increase your functional strength, increase your lean muscle mass and seriously improve the way your body takes in and utilises oxygen (cardio).

How they differ from other weight programs

The way in which we teach Kettlebells means it is a lot more than just weight loss, strength & fitness – it is also about functional movement. Static weight benches are great for 'cosmetic athletes' but don't really help to improve overall flexibility and coordination. What we are concerned about is 'functional strength'. Functional movements are movements based on real-world biomechanics. They usually involve multi-planar/ multi-joint movements which place demand on the body's core muscular system. By teaching your body to function and move the way it was intended, Kettlebells delivers results which can both be seen and felt. As Master Instructor Brett Jones says: "You can't fire a canon from a canoe".

The Performance Pyramid

The performance pyramid is a simple diagram *(below)* constructed by orthopaedic specialist and author, Gary Cook, to give you a mental image and understanding of human movement and movement patterns. It is constructed of three (3) rectangles of diminishing size, with one rectangle building upon another. Each of these rectangles represents a certain type of movement.

The first rectangular pillar is the base platform or foundation. It represents the ability to move through fundamental patterns. The second rectangular pillar is concerned with performance. Once you have established your ability to move, you must look at how efficient you are at that movement. This movement efficiency is defined as power. This is not your specific power; this is your general, measurable power (or gross athleticism). It is very important from a training standpoint to be able to compare individuals of different sports in a general format. The first two rectangular pillars allow us to make this comparison of functional movement ability and power, so that athletes can learn from each other and different training regimes. Moreover, it is important not to get sports-specific with testing at this level of the performance pyramid. Sport-specificity at this point of testing will reduce the ability to compare one athlete to another and to learn from them. It is also important not to do too many tests at this level. The more tests you do, the more you complicate matters. A few simple movements will let you know how efficient the athlete is at generating power.

The last pillar of the pyramid is sport specific skill. This pillar constitutes a battery of tests to assess the athlete's ability to do a given activity, play a specific sport, or a specific position within that sport. It looks at the competition statistics and any specific testing relative to that sport

The Performance Pyramid

As described by Gray Cook / Functional Movement Systems

What is MVO2?

O2 max (also maximal oxygen consumption, maximal oxygen uptake, peak oxygen uptake or aerobic capacity) is the maximum capacity of an individual's body to transport and use oxygen during incremental exercise, which reflects the physical fitness of the individual. The name is derived from V - volume per time, O2 - oxygen, max - maximum.

The Vo2 Max Protocol for Kettlebells is taken from Kenneth Jay, who literally wrote the book on Vo2 Max training and Kettlebells, called Viking Warrior Conditioning. In this tome of fitness written by a guy also known as the "Dane of Pain", Kenneth details his research in developing what Pavel Tsatsouline (the founder of modern Kettlebell training) calls, "a fool proof blueprint for achieving Olympian conditioning in record time - while simultaneously improving one's body composition dramatically."

A scientific assessment of the Kettlebell MVO2 protocol was undertaken in the USA. The results of that test showed the following:

> The average calorie burn was 272 calories, but that doesn't take into account the calorie burn that comes from the "substantial anaerobic effort."

> Aerobically, the subjects were burning 13.6 calories, but anaerobically, they were burning an additional 6.6 calories, which adds up to 20.2 calories per minute! (1212 calories in the hour)

According to Dr. Porcari who ran the assessment, "That's equivalent to running a 6-minute mile pace (1.6km in 6 minutes/ 10.6km/h). The only other thing I could find that burns that many calories is cross country skiing uphill at a fast pace."

Keep in mind, top marathon runners are about at a 5 and a half-minute mile.

The researchers say that the big reason for these dramatic results is because the Kettlebell snatch is a whole-body exercise that is performed with great speed and power. It is also done in an interval style which has always been an effective method of training.

The study also showed that the trainees were working at an average heart rate of 93% of maximum.

Activity	59kg	70Kg
Kettlebells MVO2	1212	
Aerobics, general	384	457
Aerobics, high impact	413	493
Aerobics, low impact	295	352
Aerobics, step aerobics	502	598
Ballet, twist, jazz, tap	266	317
Ballroom dancing, fast	325	387
Basketball game, competitive	472	563
Basketball, playing, non-game	354	422
Boxing, in ring	708	844
Boxing, punching bag	354	422
Boxing, sparring	531	633
Calisthenics, light, push-ups, sit-	207	246
Calisthenics, fast, pushes, sit-ups…	472	563
Cross country skiing, racing	826	985
Cross country skiing, uphill	974	1161
Cycling, 16-19mph, very fast, racing	708	844
Cycling, mountain bike, box	502	598
Football, competitive	531	633
Forestry, axe chopping, fast	1003	1196
Golf, walking and pulling clubs	254	303
Golf, walking and carrying clubs	266	317

What is Central Governor?

The central governor is a proposed process in the brain that regulates exercise in regard to a neurally calculated safe exertion by the body. In particular, physical activity is controlled so that its intensity cannot threaten the body's homeostasis by causing anoxia damage to the heart. The central governor limits exercise by reducing the neural recruitment of muscle fibres. This reduced recruitment is experienced as fatigue. The existence of a central governor was suggested to explain fatigue after prolonged strenuous exercise in marathons and other endurance sports, but its ideas could also apply to other causes of exertion fatigue.

Tim Noakes, a professor of exercise and sports science at the University of Cape Town: "The power output by muscles during exercise is continuously adjusted in regard to calculations made by the brain in regard to a safe level of exertion. These neural calculations factor in earlier experience with strenuous exercise, the planning duration of the exercise, and the present metabolic state of the body. These brain models ensure that body homeostasis is protected, and an emergency reserve margin is maintained. This neural control adjusts the number of activated skeletal muscle motor units, a control which is subjectively experienced as fatigue. This process, though occurring in the brain, is outside personal control."

So, to sum it up, when your body goes into fatigue (feels tired and tries to prevent you from finishing that extra set), you can actually push through by realising what your body is doing. Your body is a machine and by using your mind to battle through the fatigue, you are able to finish that set you didn't think you could. Remember, it is mind over matter. The human body is designed to withstand strenuous exercise.

<u>KB TECHNIQUES</u>

What follows are a few of the basic techniques with notes. It is recommended that this section of notes be studied in depth prior to any certification being attempted. Candidates are required to explain, teach and demonstrate these techniques. More importantly candidates must be able to correct bad technique in order to prevent injury.

Darryl Grauman

Functional Movement Basics

Deadlift

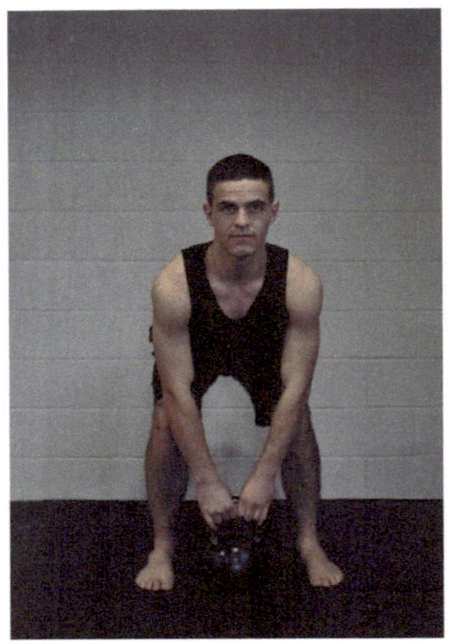

Base position, feet planted,
toes positioned forward,
knees and toes in alignment

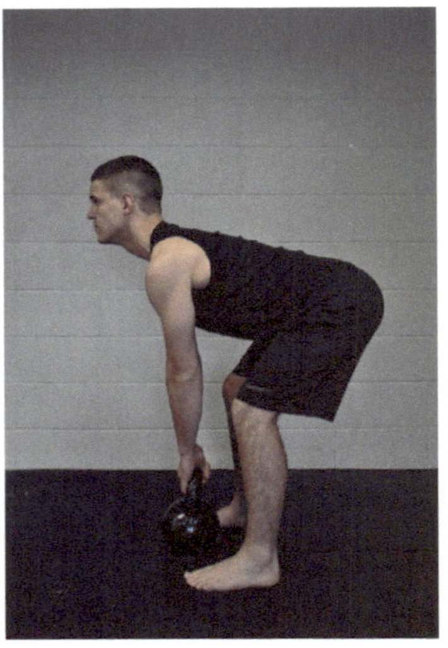

Straight back, looking forward

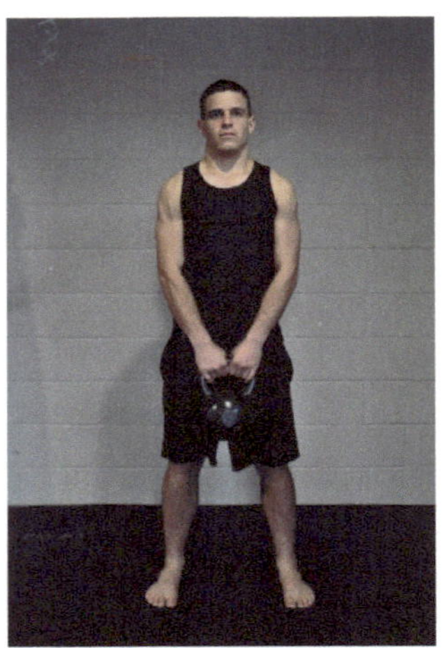

Shoulders in position and lift

Goblet Squat

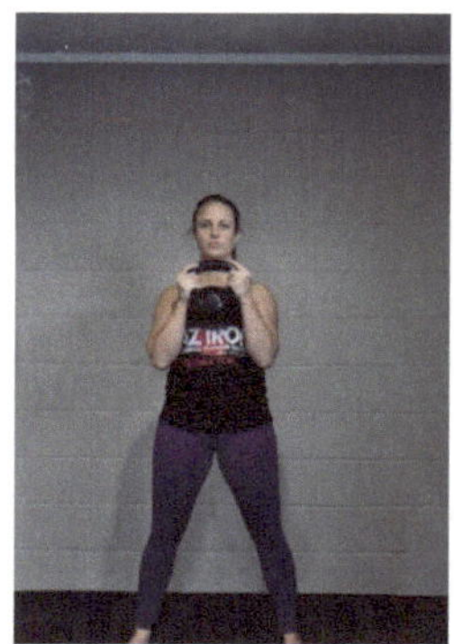

Hold KB by the horns while keeping core stability throughout

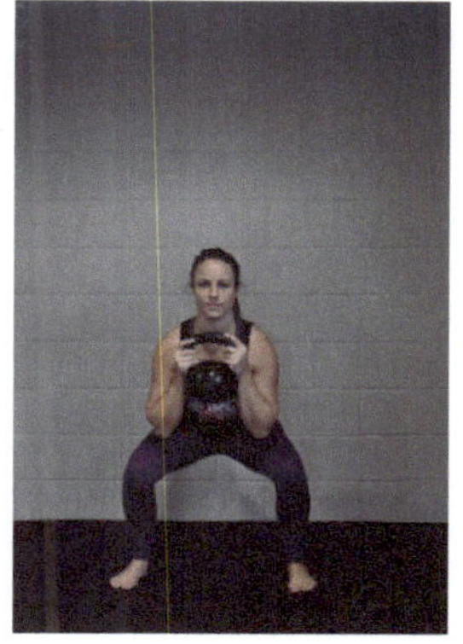

Knees and toes in alignment, begin the downward squat movement

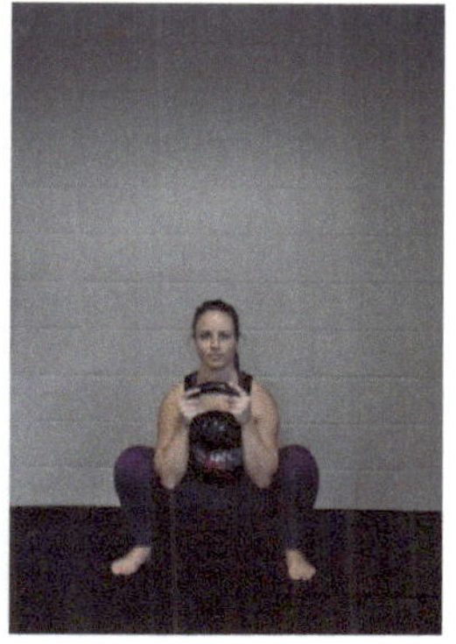

Finish the downward move looking forwards with your elbows in-between your knees and feet flat on the floor.

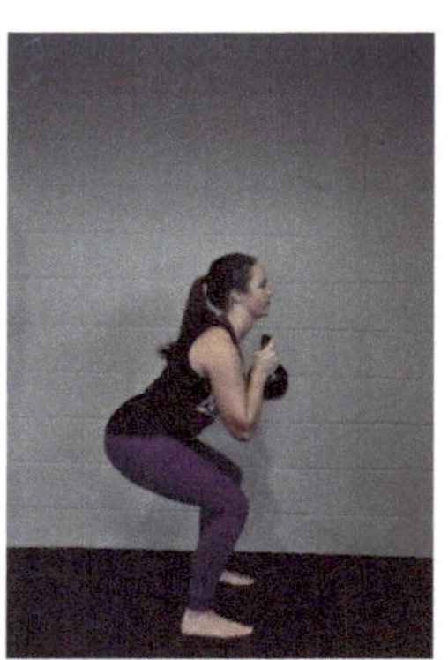

Side View, note the position of the back and that feet are still flat on the floor

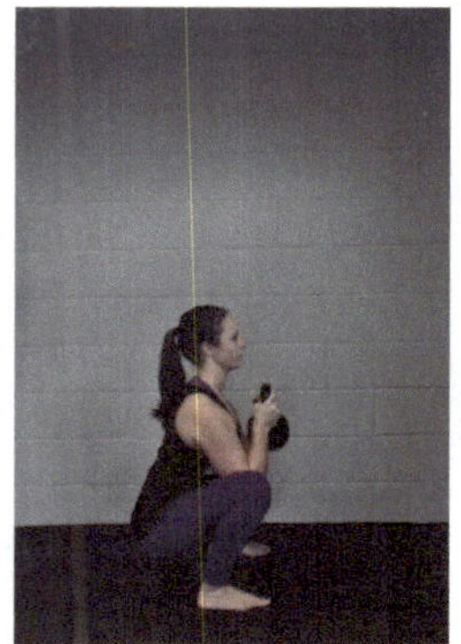

Top View - note feet and knees are straight and parallel

The Swing

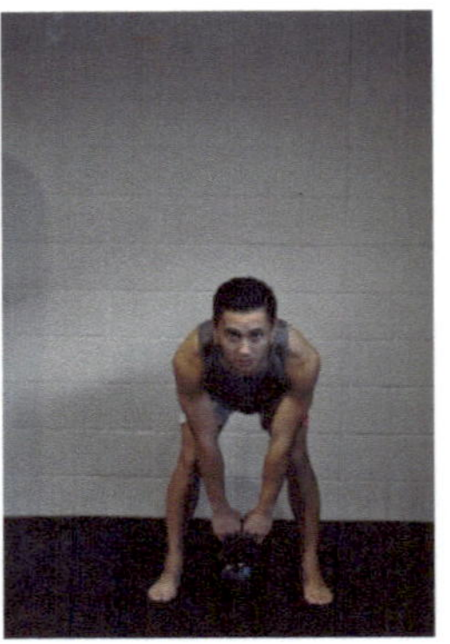

Begin in the same position
as you would a deadlift.

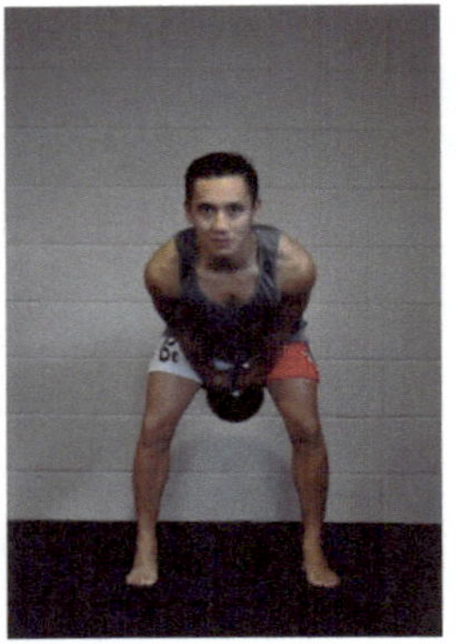

Hike the bell backwards,
while ensuring the
weight distribution on
your feet is correct and
that you do NOT rock
onto your toes.

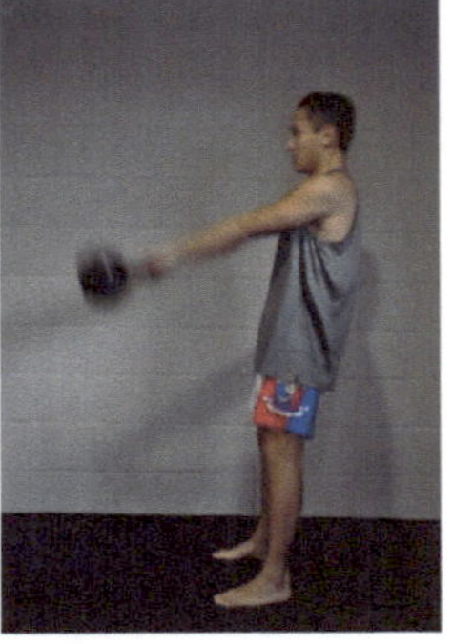

Use the ballistic
power of your legs
and your hips to
elevate the bell .

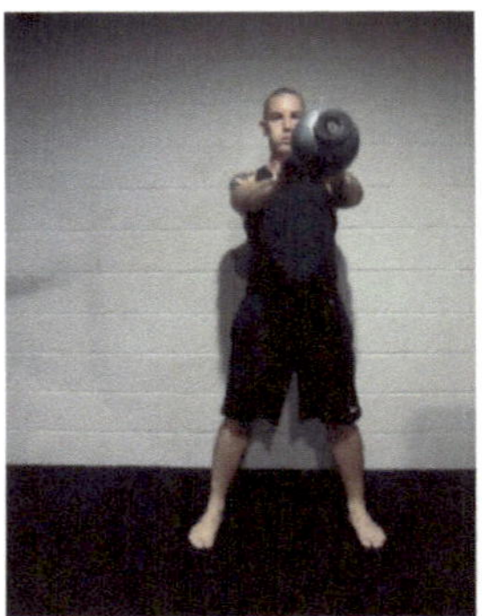

Allow the bell to swing upwards until
it swings to just about eye-level when
you employ the hardstyle lock and
downward swing.

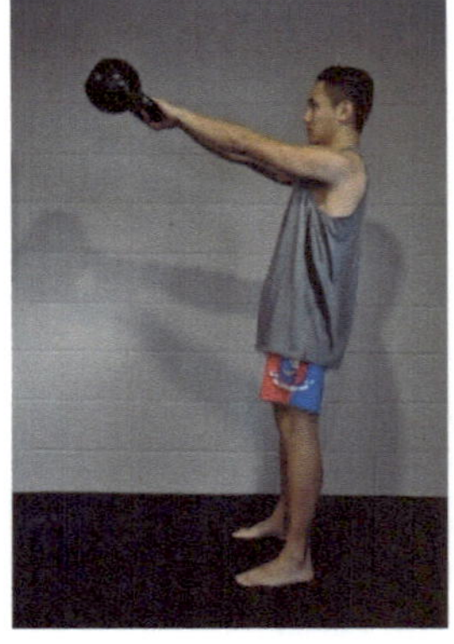

In the side view you can see how the
ballistic lift of the bell carries it
upwards as the hardstyle lock is
employed and downward swing
begins.

WARNING: See how the back remains straight! Do not lean backwards! Ensure you employ your abdominal muscles and tighten your gluteus at the top of the swing, to ensure no lean back and no back injuries!

<u>Clean</u>

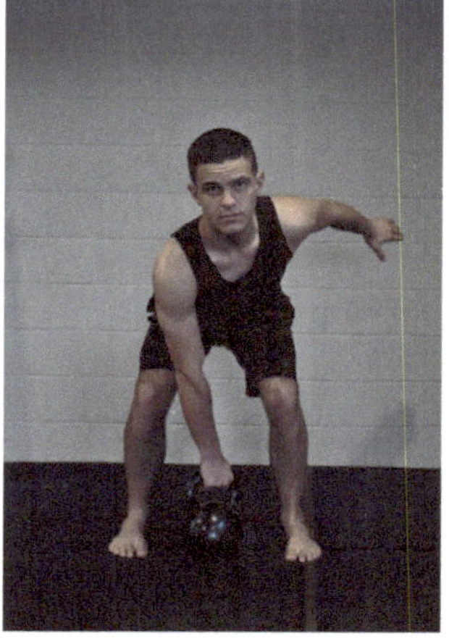

From the base deadlift stance, hike the bell downwards in a one-arm swing

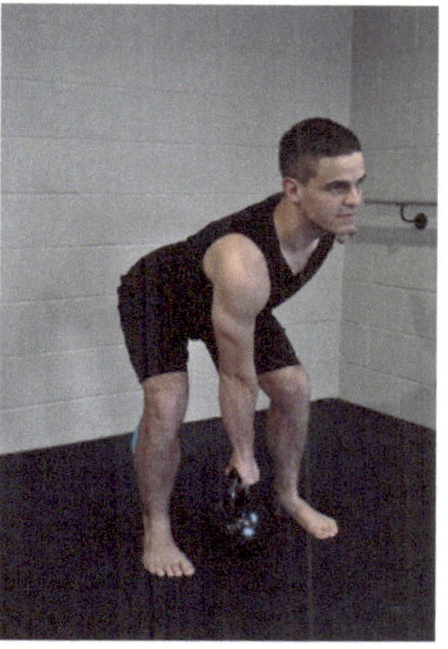

Make sure that the thumb is pointing backwards as the bell moves backwards between the legs, this ensures no shoulder injuries

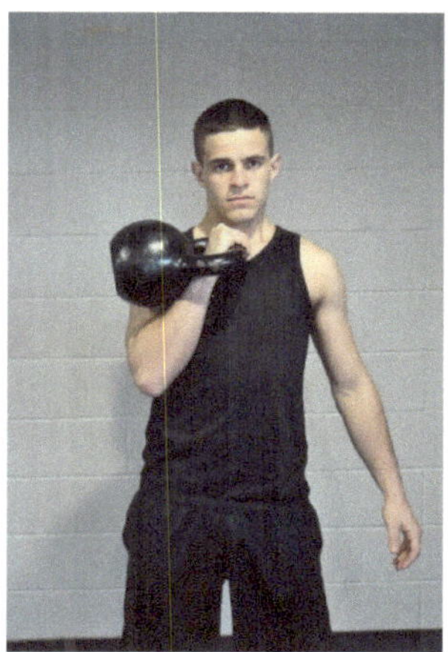

The bell is cleaned to the outside of the forearm with the core completely stable.

<u>Bicep Curl</u>

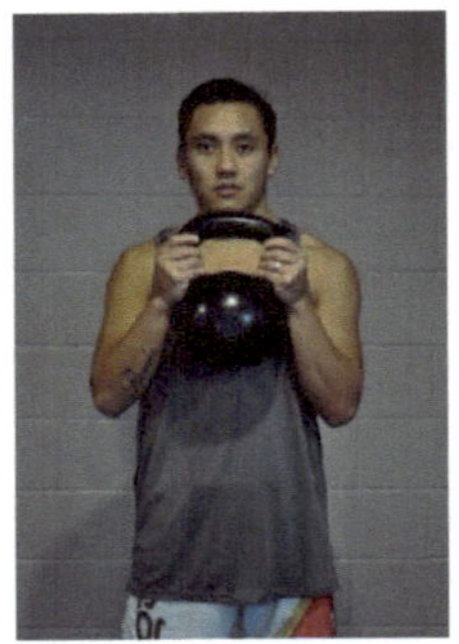

Hold the bell by the
horns

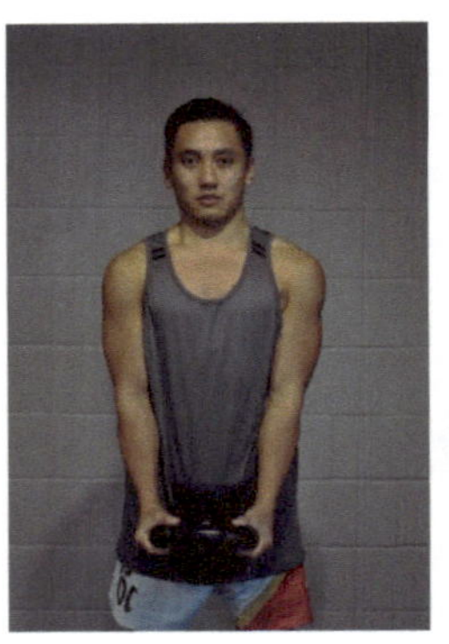

Keep your elbows
straight when you begin
this exercise

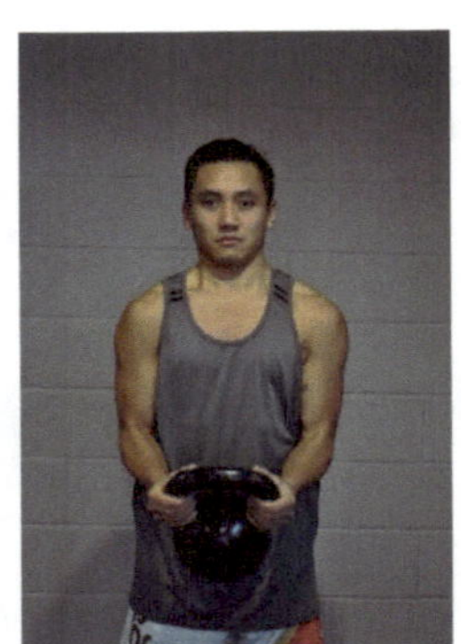

Keep your core
engaged and your
elbows close to your
sides as you lift the bell
upwards

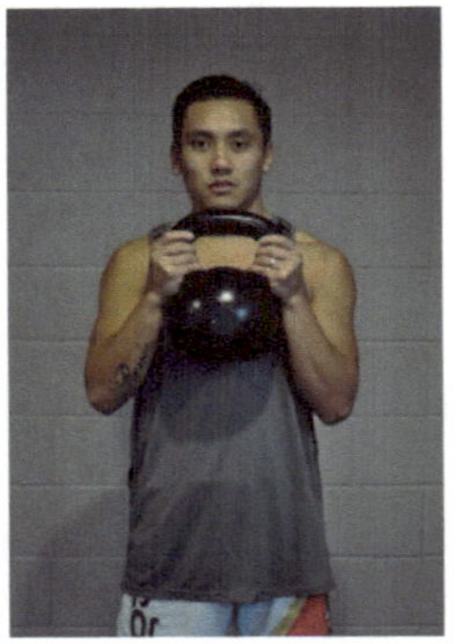

Continue to raise the
bell to just beneath your
chin. Please do not hit
yourself in the chin with
the bell!

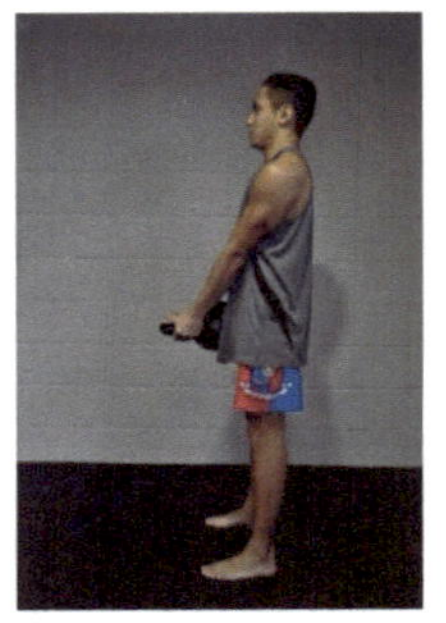

Side View, note how the
back is NOT bent!

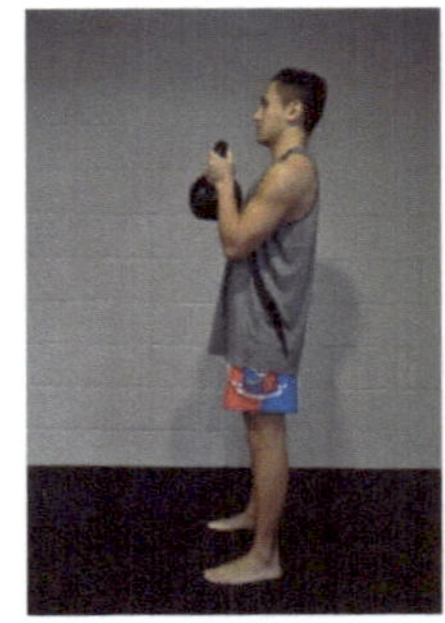

Functional Movement Intermediate

1-Arm Swing

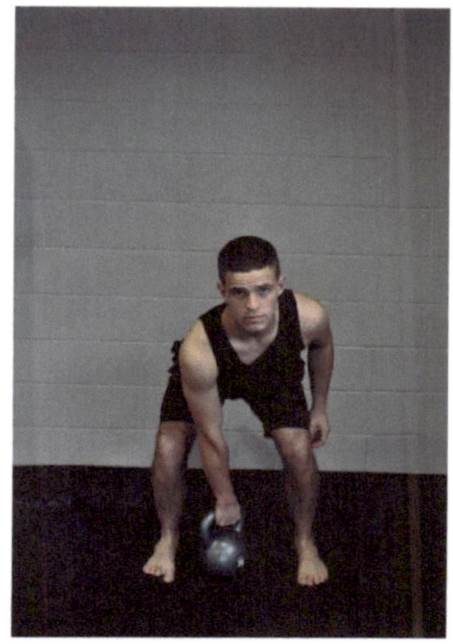

Position the bell with your thumb pointed toward you

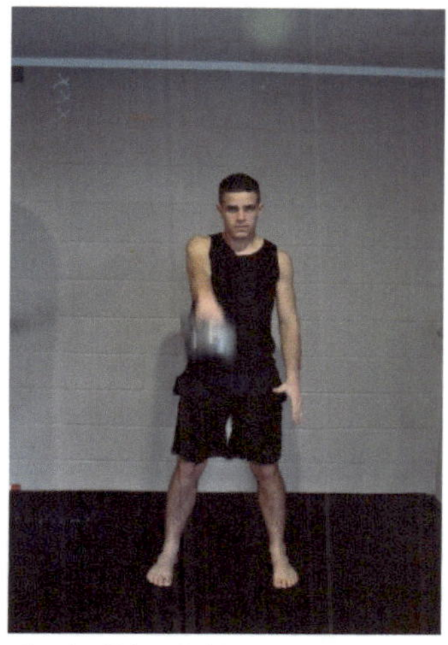

Hike the bell back like the 2-hand swing and then, using the ballistic movement of your legs and hips, elevate the bell

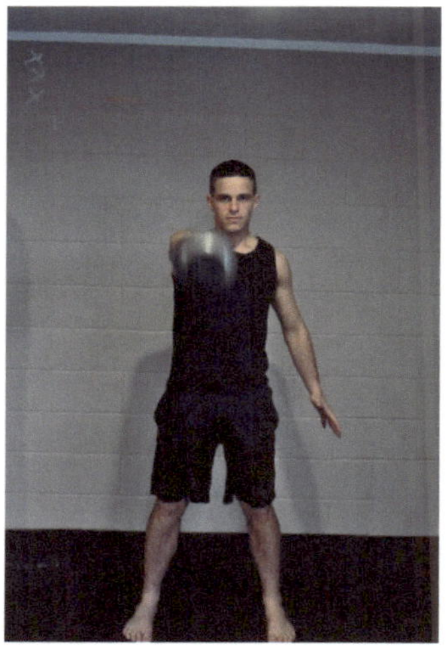

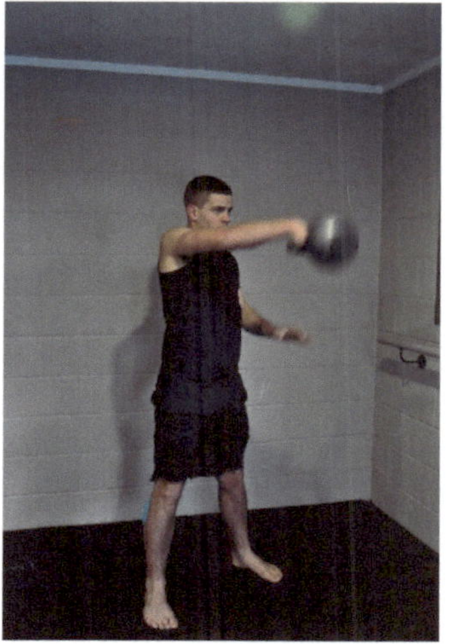

Allow the bell to swing upwards until it swings to just about eye-level when you employ the hardstyle lock and downward swing

Clean & Press

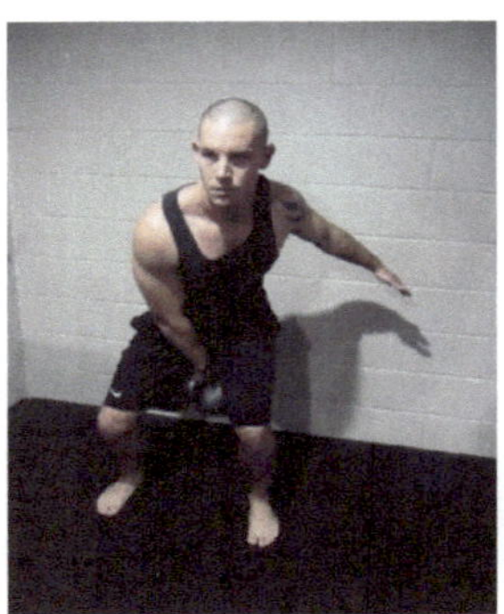

Hike the bell similar to a one arm swing

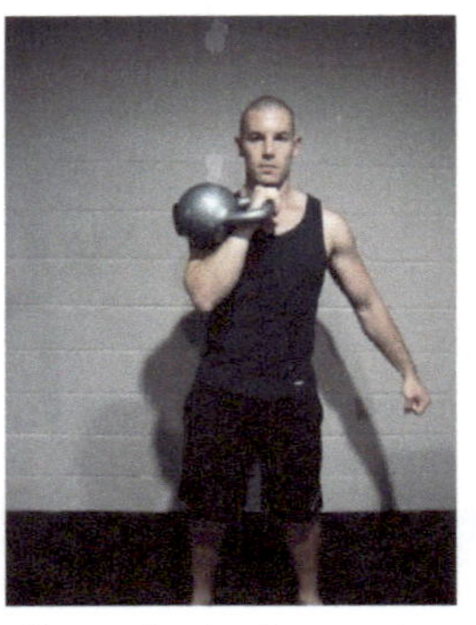

Clean the bell ensuring a completely stabile core

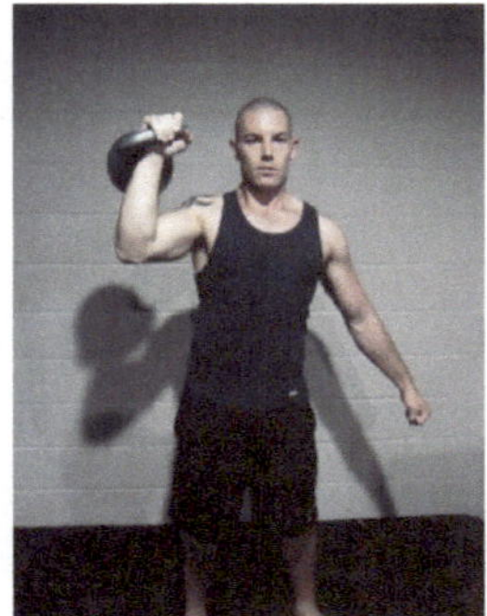

A knee bend can be employed at this time.

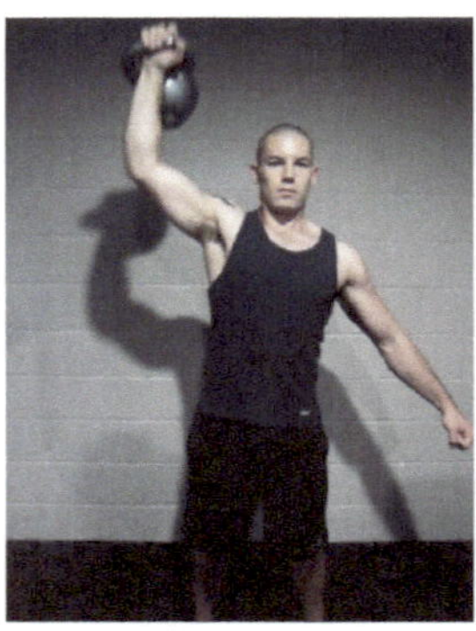

Press the bell towards the sky ensuring a completely stabile core

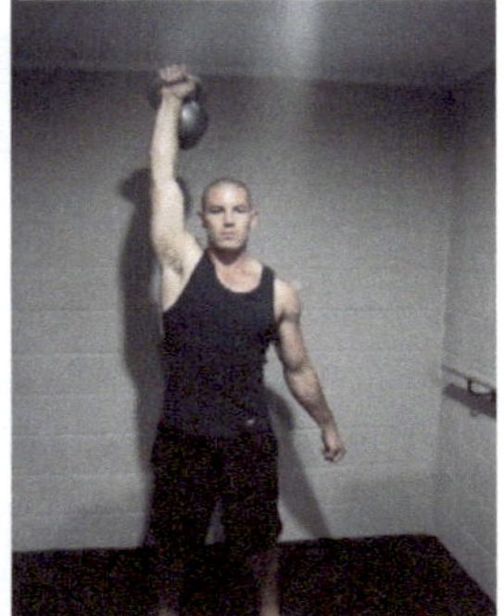

Finish in the lockout position with entire core engaged.

WARNING:

See how the back remains straight! Do not lean backwards! Ensure you employ your abdominal muscles and tighten your gluteus at the top of the swing, to ensure no lean back and no back injuries!

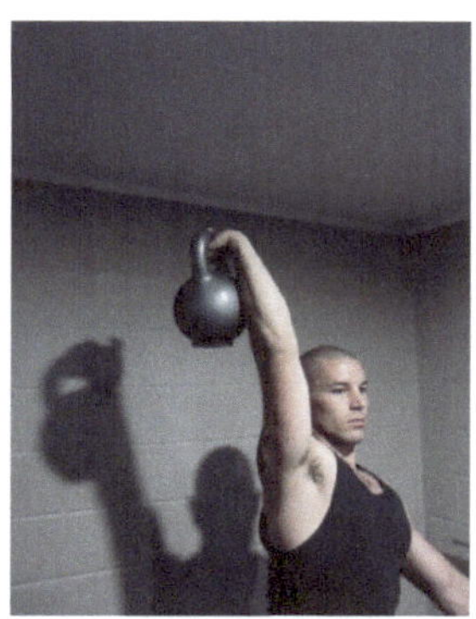

Keep your wrist straight
and do not allow the bell
to drift behind your ear
**Do NOT bend your
wrist!**

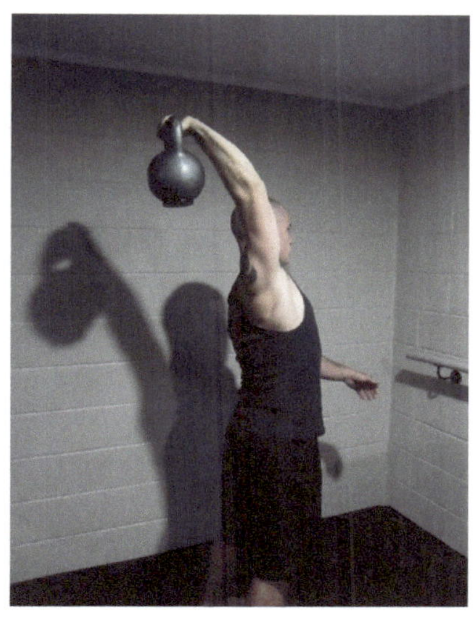

**Be CAREFUL not to extend the bell too far
behind the ear**

Alternating Swing

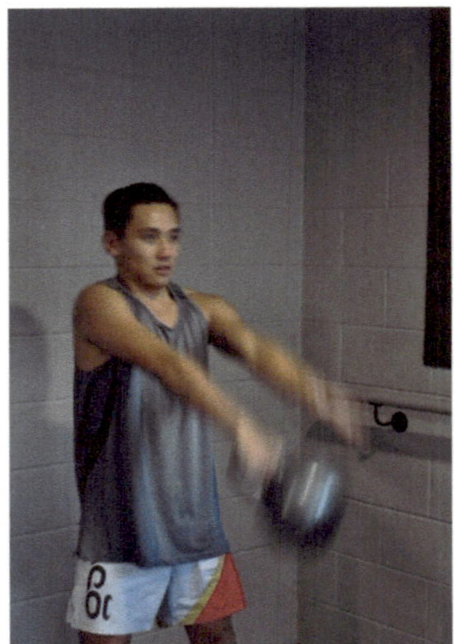

Begin as if you are doing a 1-arm swing

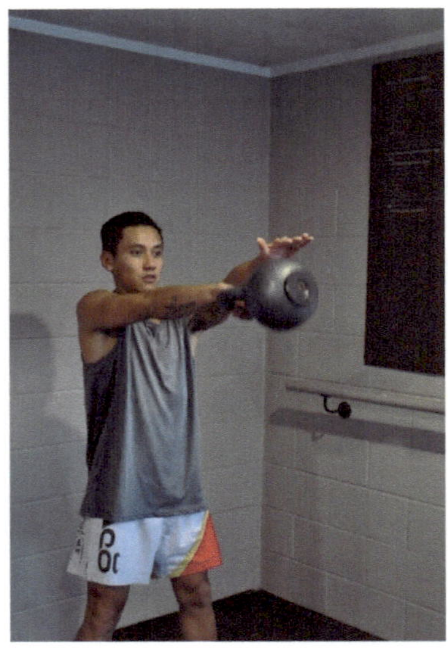

As the bell is about to reach the apex just in front of your chin be prepared for a hand change

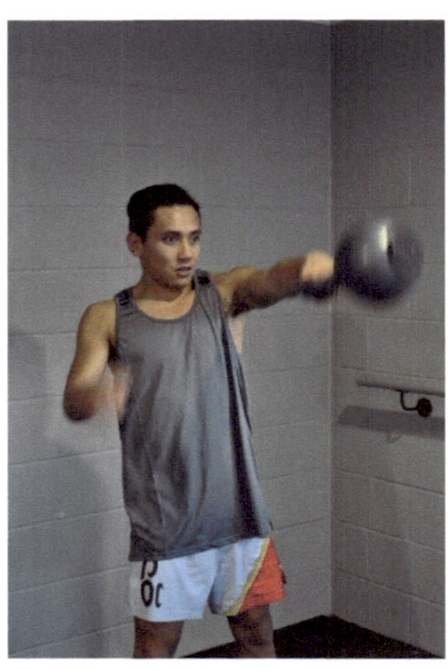

Firmly execute a hand change without letting the bell out of your control!
Please be careful and do not attempt this for the first time with people in front of you!

Snatch

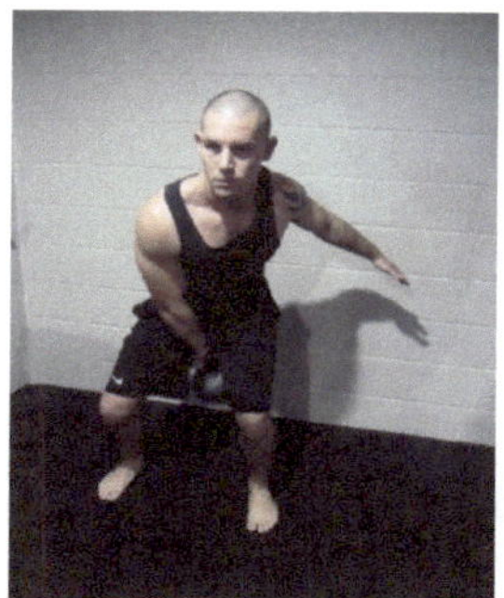

Hike the bell similar to a one arm swing

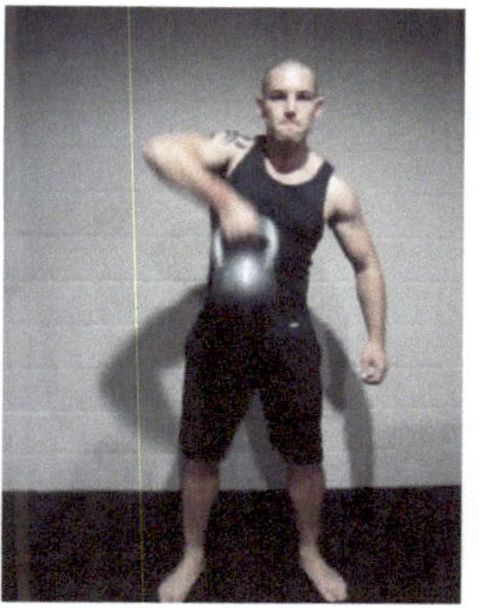

Use the ballistic power of your legs to bring the bell upwards with a bent elbow almost centreline with your body

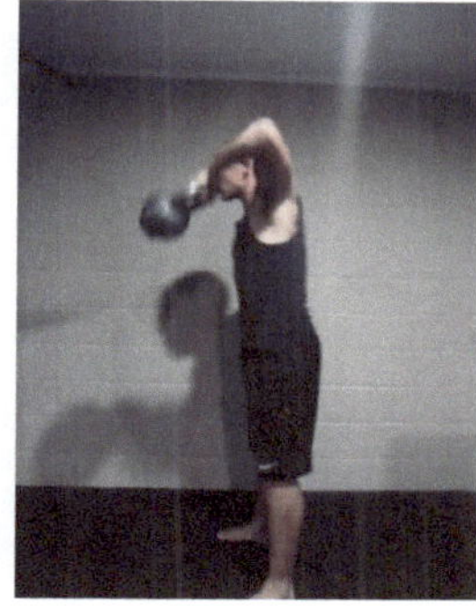

Notice how the bell is brought upwards with a bent elbow and flat palm

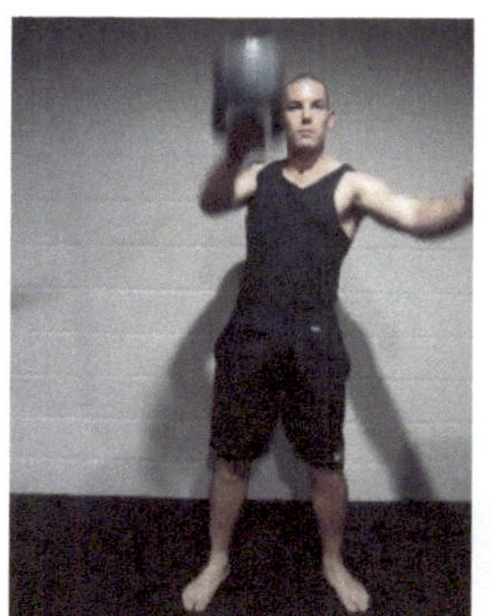

The snatch is competed when you "punch" out into the snatch position and the bell comes to rest gently on your forearm

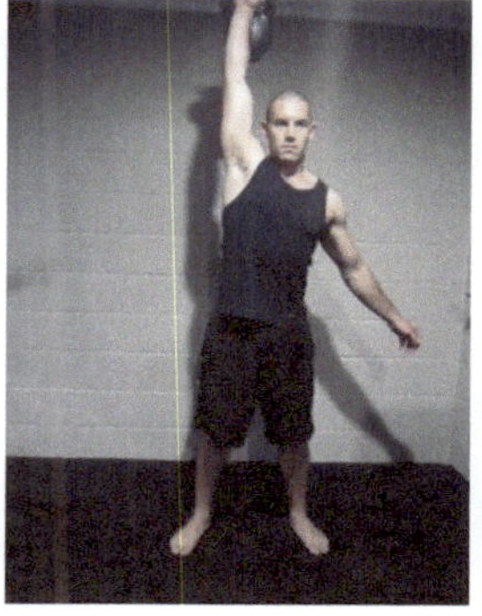

Finish in the lockout position with abdominals and gluteus engaged

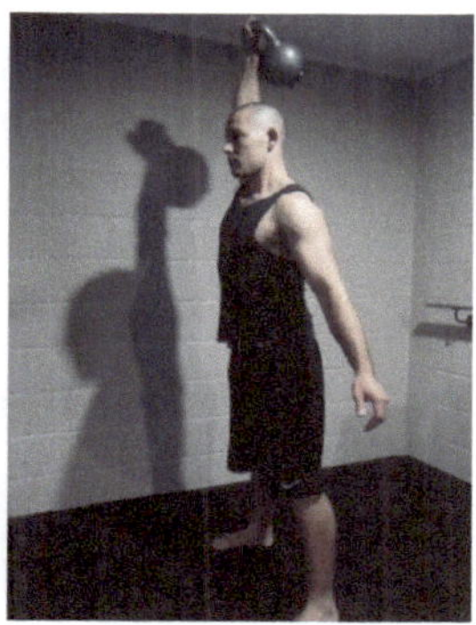

Note the lockout and body alignment

Military Press

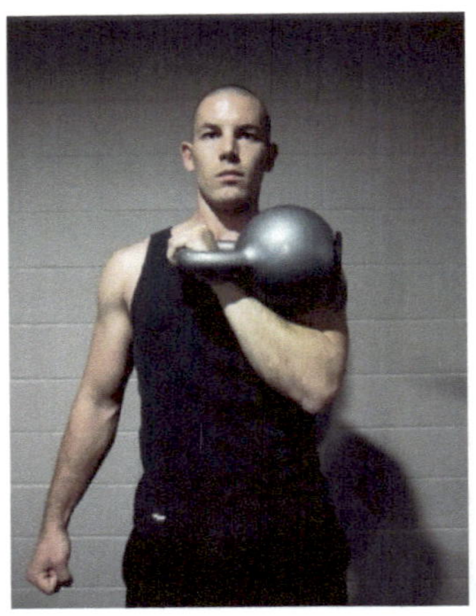

Clean the bell and bring it in to your chest while ensuring your core is engaged and the bell is resting on the heel of your hand

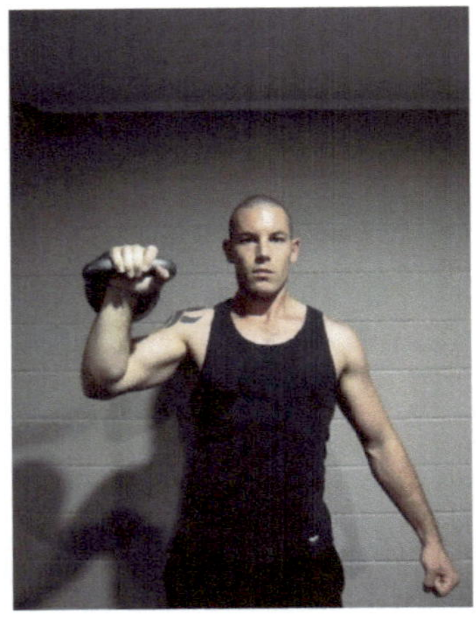

With your feet planted firmly and your core engaged, begin to press the bell towards the sky. Imagine the heel of your hand against the top of a door frame and you are trying to push away

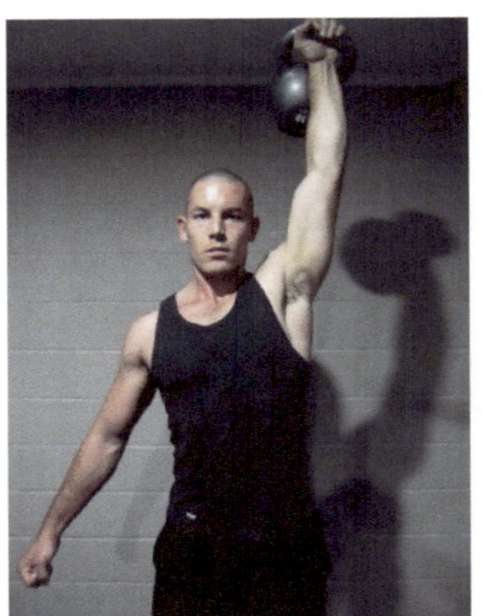

End with a complete lockout with abdominals and gluteus engaged

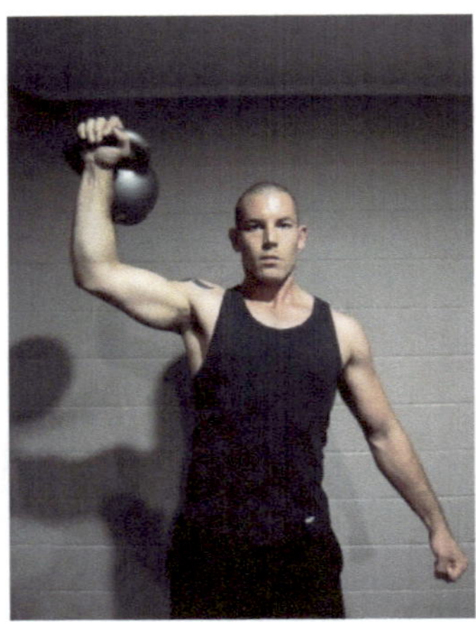

Engage and "flare" the latissimus dorsi (lats) as you bring the bell down into the start position.

<u>2-Hand Upright Row</u>

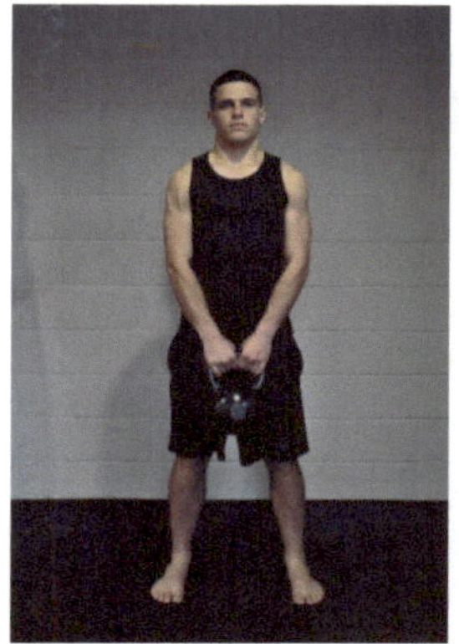 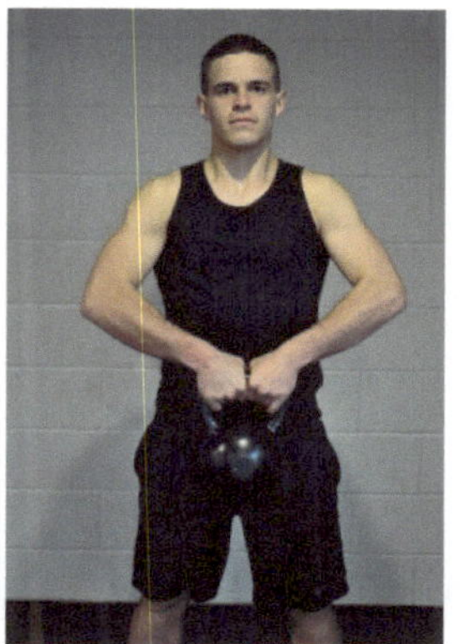 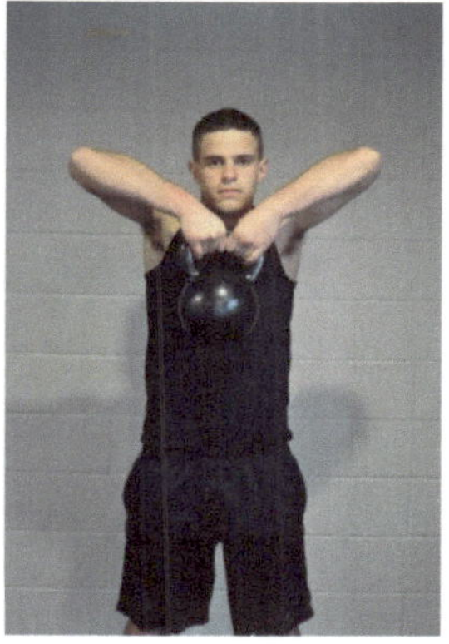

| Hold the bell as if you have just completed a deadlift | With your core engaged, raise the bell toward your chin by raising your elbows toward the sky | Finish with your elbows high and the bell just under your chin. Control the bell downwards to the start position. |

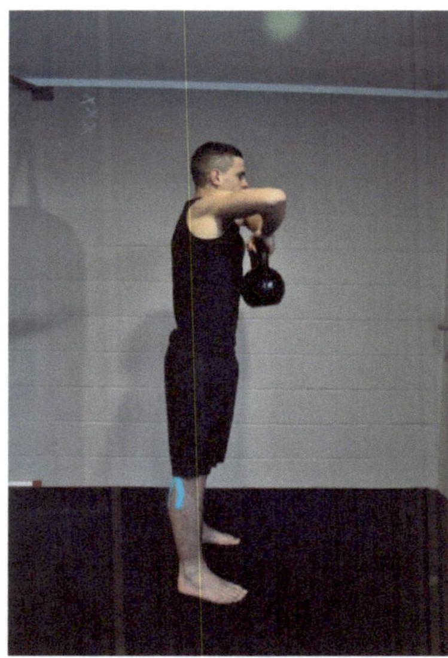

Once again note how the abdominals and glutes are engaged, keeping the back straight.

TRAINING AIDS FOR PERSONAL TRAINERS

VO2Max Cadence Test
(Credit: Dr Kenneth Jay, Viking Warrior Conditioning)

Snatch Cadence Test:
- 1st Minute - 10 reps or 1 rep per 6 seconds
- 2nd Minute - 14 reps or 1 rep per 4.2 seconds
- 3rd Minute - 18 reps or 1 rep per 3.3 seconds
- 4th Minute - 22 reps or 1 rep per 2.7 seconds
- 5th minute - all out, as many reps as possible. (Count them!).

The last minute = Your cVO2 Max, the cadence that elicits a VO2 Max response.

- If you achieve 24 reps or less in 5th minute, pick up a <u>lighter</u> bell and do it again in 15 minutes time.

- If you achieve 40 reps or more in 5th minute, pick up a <u>heavier</u> bell and do it again in 15 minutes time.

To get your number of repetitions for the 15:15 VO2Max, divide your 1 minute cadence by 4 and round up! E.g.: if you achieved 26 reps in the last minute, the formula would be:
- 26 / 4 = 6.5
- Round up = 7 reps every 15 seconds

Training Diary

Food Diary (for 12 weeks)

Now you don't need to go counting calories but it is a good idea to keep track of what your clients are consuming so you are aware of their energy intake. You should pay attention to what they are consuming and at what times of the day. In the back of this manual is an example of a food diary. We suggest that for at least the first 3-4 weeks of a training program you use this diary to record EVERYTHING that passes your clients lips!

Why do people get fat?

If you received three of the same body lotions for your birthday what would you do? You could give one away, recycle as a gift or store it so you can use it in the future. Fat is like that body lotion sitting at the back of your bathroom cupboard that you never use. You keep buying new ones because you're sick of that same lotion so it continues to sit there. Fat is the same in that your body will store excess energy which it cannot use. We get our energy from food and drink so if we continue to consume high-energy food and drink regularly, the stored fat will stay and accumulate.

Unfortunately losing the stored fat is not as easy as doing a bathroom clean up. The energy consumed must be less than the energy required for your body to function normally but this must be done in a safe and healthy way in order for your body to cope with weight loss. Exercise can help with weight loss but 80% of weight loss is your nutrition.

Why you get a six-pack in the kitchen, not the gym

There is an old bodybuilding adage that states, "Great abs are made in the kitchen, not in the gym." It's a catchy little saying and when I say it, most people pause and then say, "Oh, I get it!" After all, it's a really simple concept. Another way of conveying this truth is "you can't out exercise a bad diet." Consider this common example: Julie is a woman of average height and weight that goes to the gym with her friends. Feeling strong one day, she decides to push it on the treadmill at 6 mph for an entire hour. One sweaty hard worked hour later she looks down and the treadmill reads "Calories Burned: 661." "Sweeeet!" she says. Feeling fantastic, Julie and her friends decide to grab a bite to eat and hang out for a bit before heading home. They decide to go to their favourite local deli and get something "light" since they are in that healthy frame of mind. Julie orders her favourite bagel with light cream cheese and a small fruit smoothie.

Riding on her exercise high, Julie enjoys her bagel and smoothie while visiting with her friends. As their lunch is winding down and realizing they still have a lot to do that day, the girls decide to grab a quick "pick-me-up" to head into the second half of the day. It's hot outside so Julie orders her favourite ice-blended coffee drink with light milk and heads home. Entering her house, she tosses her keys on the counter, drops her empty coffee cup into the recycling bin and heads into the shower.

This is where we need to press pause in our little story. Something has happened. Little does she know it, but Julie has already consumed more calories in that quick trip to the deli and coffee shop than she burned in that sweaty one-hour workout at the gym! That is how quickly it happens.

- Bagel: 320 calories
- Light Cream Cheese: 100 calories
- Fruit Smoothie: 240 calories
- Blended Mocha: 280 calories
- Total Calories: 940

And you can add another 100-200 calories to that total if she chugged down a sports drink while exercising. It's a difficult thing to digest (pun intended) but it's a vital thing to truly understand if we are going to educate ourselves on the process of shedding unwanted pounds.

Along with the above example, there is something of equal importance to understand when it comes to getting those ripped 6-pack abs. YOU ALREADY HAVE THEM! We all do, anatomically speaking. It's just a matter of making them visible. As evidence to this, just spend a little time at your local municipal pool and you will see droves of kids walking around with perfect 6-pack abs who have never done a crunch in their life! So often in training sessions you will hear a person say, while clutching a piece of their belly fat, "Can we do a lot of abs today, because I gotta get rid of this." This is a misnomer, though common to all trainers, which has persisted in the public eye for years.

The majority of the reason for this is that whenever we are shown someone in a fitness magazine or TV spot discussing how to get those ripped abs, they are typically doing some sort of abdominal exercise or using some type of equipment they want to sell you. The marketing process is simple. Show someone with great abs using a product and the consumer ties the image of great abs to the use of that product. And it works. The sales of ab equipment are a multi-million-dollar business. **But the truth lies in your refrigerator.**

<u>Your Goals & Measurements Diary</u>

Your Realistic Goals:

1. ______________________________________

   ____

2. ______________________________________

   ____

Your Personal Tracker:

	Weight	Hips	Tummy	Chest	Upper Arms
Week 0 - Let's Go!					
Week 3					
Week 6					
Week 9					
Week 12 – Woohoo!					

MVO2 Accomplishment Diary

(Protocol x KB weight x reps per period x sets)

Date	MVO2 Description	Kettlebell Weight	Reps per Phase	Total Sets
E.g.: 1/1/2015	15:15 Protocol	12kg	7	60

Functional Movement Screen Results

Date	Deep Squat	Hurdle Step	In-Line Lunge	Shoulder Mobility	Active Straight Leg Raise	Trunk Stability Pushup	Rotational Stability	Total

Appendix: Food Diary

	Monday	Tuesday	Wednesday	Thursday	Friday	Saturday	Sunday
Pre-Workout							
Post Workout							
Breakfast							
Morning Snack							
Lunch							
Afternoon Snack							
Pre-Workout							
Post Workout							
Dinner							
Water							
Coffee							
Alcohol							
Exercise							

Reflect on Your Day

Circle Y for Yes and N for No

- Did you eat something today only because of habit? Y / N
- Did you skip any meals today? Y / N
- Did you go longer than four to five hours without eating? Y / N
- Did you eat too little in the morning? Y / N
- Did you eat more at night than any other time? Y / N
- Did you eat a lot of high-fat foods, such as whole dairy, fried foods, and desserts? Y / N
- Did you eat the same foods as you do every other day? Y / N
- Did you eat according to mood rather than hunger today? Y / N

<u>NZ Iron Instructor Certification Requirements</u>

*Please note that the requirements described below are subject to change

You may choose to attend a NZ Iron course even if you are not intending to teach. Meaning that if you are taking the course for personal development and forgo the testing phase you will

The following comprise overall certification requirements for Level 1 (Beginner/Intermediate):

- Awareness of the concepts and practices of Functional Movement
- Understanding of the MVO2 & "Viking Warrior Conditioning" concepts
- Complete the full 1 Hour prescribed workout on each day of the course
  - Day 1: Functional Movement Set 1, 2 & 3 (upper body, abdominals, legs)
  - Day 2: 80-Set Mixed MVO2
- Pass the Snatch test that will be administered at the examination date or on the last day of the course
- Demonstrate personal mastery of the techniques contained in the course manual
- Demonstrate an ability to teach all of the techniques contained in the course manual to a novice
- Demonstrate a good understanding of Kettlebell safety
- Demonstrate an understanding of the difference in instruction between one-on-one training and group classes
- Follow the NZ Iron Code of Conduct

Testing Requirement

Day 1 & Day 2 Functional Movement Sets and Mixed MVO2 will be taught and executed on each of the days. Participants need to complete both workouts to the end.

NZ Iron candidates must also pass a further conditioning test to assess their cardiovascular, strength and endurance conditioning. The Kettlebell snatch test is the definitive test for the candidate's technique under stress (timed) conditions.

The candidate should wear clothing that does not restrict movement not restrict the examiners view of the technique. Please inform your instructors if you have any injuries which would prevent you from demonstrating clear and proper technique.

Gloves and hand wraps are acceptable for the test, although bare hand is preferred. Chalk may be used and re-applied at any time during the test. No other body support apparatus such as weight belts will be allowed.

Snatch Test

Begin with the Kettlebell at your feet and prepare for the signal to begin. Snatch the Kettlebell overhead in one movement, ending with a straight-arm lock out. The instructor will count the repetitions for only those where proper lock-out technique is demonstrated.

- You may swing and change hands as required
- You may set the Kettlebell down and rest as required
- A timer will be within sight and timer counts will be provided by the instructor

A no count will be given if:

- Elbows are not locked at the top of the snatch
- Abdominal and gluteus maximus muscles are not locked at the top of the snatch
- Knees are re-bent on the way up

- Heels come up off the floor
- Failure to stop all movement at the lockout
- Pressing the Kettlebell to finish the lockout
- Passing the snatch hand through the rack position on the way down

Immediate failure will occur if the candidate
- Has three no counts in a row
- Drops the Kettlebell so that it hits the ground with force
- Runs out of time before completing the required number of repetitions

Technique Tests:

As a NZ Iron instructor you will need to demonstrate proper and safe technique. The following are techniques that will be tested either on the last day of the course or during the exam at a later date:
- Deadlift
- Goblet Squat
- 2-Arm Swing
- 1-Arm Swing
- Clean
- Clean & Press
- Military Press
- High Pull
- Snatch

Non-Tested Techniques:

A number of techniques will be taught on this course but are not tested at this level; they include, but are not limited to:
- Single-Leg Deadlifts
- Farmers Carries
- Kettlebell Lunges
- Windmills

- Turkish Get-up
- 2-Hand Upright Rows
- Bicep Curl
- Renegade Rows
- Pullover Sit-up
- Kettlebell Stand-up

Teaching Requirements:

During the testing phase you will be asked to demonstrate your ability to teach any of the above techniques to a Kettlebell novice. You will have 30 minutes to privately train your "student" using the techniques and progressions you learned on the course. This instruction may be observed by your examiner. After the 30 minutes the "student" will be asked to demonstrate the techniques to the examiner.
Your evaluation will be based on how efficiently and effectively you taught the techniques and implemented any corrections to improper technique.

If you a fail a requirement:

Should you fail to make the requirements during the official test, you may arrange to be re-tested. You have 3 months to retest the section(s) that you failed. Please contact info@nziron.co.nz to arrange either a video or personal re-test. A fee may be applicable. You also have the option to retake the course within one year, for which the fee to attend is $200.

The NZ Iron Code of Conduct

NZ Iron is an organisation based on professional and physical principles; the people representing NZ Iron are the true face of the organisation and the way the organisation is perceived by the public and the fitness industry as a whole.

To this end we would look to certified NZ Iron instructors to follow the professional code of conduct below:-

As a certified NZ Iron Kettlebell Instructor, I will:

- Promote the principles and values of NZ Iron to the best of my ability through professional and moral conduct at all times including in public and through social media
- Be an ambassador of NZ Iron training through the continued refinement and learning of technique and the way I impart that to clients and other members of the public
- Know my own limitations as an instructor and will refer to other professionals as required
- Treat all of those who I teach and train with respect and humility

Failure to adhere to the above could result in a revocation of certification.

Appendix: Snatch Test Requirements:

Men:

- Up to 72kg   20kg   100/5 min
- Over 72kg   24kg   100/5 min

Men's Masters: (50-64yrs)

- Up to 65kg   16kg   100/5 min
- 65.1kg-78kg   20kg   100/5 min
- Over 78kg   24kg   100/6 min

Women:

- Up to 54kg   12kg   100/5 min
- Over 54.1kg   16kg   100/5 min

Women Masters: (50-64yrs)

- Up to 54kg   10kg   100/5 min
- 54.1-63kg   12kg   100/5min
- Over 63kg   16kg   100/5 min

NZ Iron Instructor Certification Testing Scoresheet Example:

Candidate Name: ________________

Pre-Assessment:

Topic:	Pass/ Fail	Comments:
Client understanding - Physicality		
Client Understanding – Injuries / Impediments		
Client Understanding - Goals		

Progressions Assessment:

Topic:	Explanation	Demonstration	Correction	Perfection	Pass/ Fail
Deadlift > Swing					
Swing > 1-Hand Swing					
1-Hand Swing > High Pull					
High Pull > Snatch					

Technique Tests:

Topic:	Explanation	Demonstration	Correction	Perfection	Pass/Fail
Deadlift					
Goblet Squat					
2-Arm Swing					
1-Arm Swing					
Clean					
Clean & Press					
Military Press					
High Pull					
Snatch					

Snatch Test

Begin with the Kettlebell at your feet and prepare for the signal to begin. Snatch the Kettlebell overhead in one movement, ending with a straight-arm lock out. The instructor will count the repetitions for only those where proper lock-out technique is demonstrated.

- You may swing and change hands as required
- You may set the Kettlebell down and rest as required
- A timer will be within sight and timer counts will be provided by the instructor

A no count will be given if:

- Elbows are not locked at the top of the snatch
- Abdominal and gluteus maximus muscles are not locked at the top of the snatch
- Knees are re-bent on the way up
- Heels come up off the floor
- Failure to stop all movement at the lockout
- Pressing the Kettlebell to finish the lockout
- Passing the snatch hand through the rack position on the way down

Immediate failure will occur if the candidate

- Has three no counts in a row
- Drops the Kettlebell so that it hits the ground with force
- Runs out of time before completing the required number of repetitions

<u>Snatch Test</u>	
Overall # Snatches Performed	
# non-counted Snatches	
Time to compete 100	
Pass/ Fail	

Darryl Grauman

Preview:

NZ Iron Level 2 Training Manual

CONTENTS

1. The Basics of Pre-Hab/Re-Hab 101
   a. Periscope
   b. Sphinx
   c. Crawling
   d. Tall Kneeling
   e. Half Kneeling
2. Double Bells:
   a. Swing
   b. Clean & Press
   c. Snatch
   d. Windmills
3. Developing a Program:
   a. Strength
   b. Cardiovascular (beyond the 15:15)
   c. Endurance
   d. Group Classes
4. Workout : MaxGains / Rounds / Double Bells

ABOUT DR MARK CHENG

Dr Mark Cheng

Since his youth, Dr. Mark Cheng developed quite a fascination with traditional martial arts. As a child, he began his foray into Chinese martial arts by learning the rudiments of self-defence and Tai-Chi with his father. The artistry, athleticism, character building, cultural pride, and self-confidence aspects he saw portrayed in East Asian cinema won him over early on, and he sought out the top instructors of many different disciplines to study with and train under when he relocated to the Los Angeles area to attend college.

During his undergraduate career, spanning from Caltech to UCLA (where he graduated with his baccalaureate in East Asian Studies), Cheng was exposed to a wide variety of martial arts styles and systems from around the world. As he researched more deeply into the Chinese martial arts, he noticed that all of the most respected masters were also well versed in Chinese tautological medicine ("Dit Da", sometimes referred to as "Chinese osteopathy") at a minimum while some even became practicing licensed acupuncturists and herbalists. In dealing with the various injuries, including muscle strains, sprains, fractures, and joint injuries, these skilled masters demonstrated the healing potential of their different acupuncture, herbal, and Tui-Na manual treatment abilities on Cheng and many others.

The treatments and their immediate benefits left such a profound impression on Cheng that he went on to earn his Masters and Doctorate (Ph.D.) degrees in Chinese medicine and acupuncture, as well as his California State acupuncture license (L.Ac.), allowing him to practice professionally. He also taught Tui-Na (Chinese manual therapeutics) for two of the strongest Chinese medicine colleges in the Los Angeles area.

Not content to rest on the strength of his coursework, Dr.

Cheng also made regular efforts to study with the top Chinese-style manual therapists, Western physical therapists, and strength training experts to gain a wider understanding of the human body and the safest, most efficient ways of helping it perform at a higher level with less pain and dysfunction.

Today, Dr. Cheng owns a successful private practice in Santa Monica, California, gives speaking engagements, workshops, & seminars internationally, and is constantly working on producing better instructional resources for improving athletic performance in elite athletes and more pain-free movement and strength for everyday people.

ABOUT THE AUTHOR

Darryl Grauman has been training in various forms of martial arts for 40 years. Darryl has a degree in psychology, law and a postgraduate business degree. By profession he works in the ICT sector running part of a multi-billion dollar, global organisation. He has a 5th Degree black belt in Ju-Jitsu, and black belts in judo and kung-fu. He has trained extensively in Catch Wrestling, Krav Maga and BJJ. He is a Chinese Kickboxing (San-Shou) coach and has produced a number of champions in NZ and overseas. Darryl has now been teaching MMA in for the last 20 years and runs the MMA, Grappling and Self Defence sessions at Redline Combat in Auckland, New Zealand. Darryl has also been training in Kettlebells under Dr Mark Cheng for many years and founded the NZ Iron Kettlebell Training organisation which helps to teach Personal Trainers, Performance Athletes and other Fitness, Physical and Medical Professionals in the safe use of kettlebells. Darryl is regarded as an authority on Kettlebells in NZ and runs intensive Kettlebell & Conditioning sessions at Redline. Darryl also consults on fight preparation for professional and amateur athletes.

Darryl's own bout with Cancer has helped refine many of the programs he teaches. Darryl used his own kettlebell programs to prepare for cancer treatment and recover post major surgery.

9 781974 036585